Self Published by Shahnawaaz Khan

Shahnawaaz Khan is a Registered Nutritionist and a Member of the Nutrition Council Australia.

This book **does not** take your individual circumstances into account, nor does it claim to cure, heal or treat any illness or medical condition.
If you are experiencing any medical/ health concerns please speak to your Doctor. The contents of this book are intended for *otherwise healthy* individuals who are seeking information about how to make healthier choices, who want to learn about the nutritional content of foods they are consuming, and their importance to the human body.

Actionable Nutrition provides guidance on how to create a Meal Plan from scratch. It may be an offence under the prevailing laws of your local area to provide Meal Plans to Friends, Family and 'Clients' for the purpose of making money. In most jurisdictions (Globally) a Licence/ Registration is required to do so.

Every effort has been made to ensure the accuracy of information provided, though things can sometimes be overlooked. Shahnawaaz Khan reserves the right to make corrections for information provided in error.

A catalogue for this book is available from the National Library of Australia (NLA) in Canberra.

Declaration: NO part of this book/ work was written/ created by the use of Generative AI.

Edited by, Shahnawaaz Khan

Paperback: ISBN 978-0-646-73351-7
Ebook: ISBN 978-0-646-71711-1

Cover Image: Canva
Book cover design by Shahnawaaz Khan

WITH THANKS TO MY FAMILY FOR THEIR CONTINUED LOVE AND SUPPORT

CHAPTER 1:

DIGESTION

BENEFITS OF A HEALTHY DIGESTIVE SYSTEM

The health of our digestive system directly impacts our overall well-being. An effectively functioning digestive system leads to numerous health benefits. An unhealthy digestive system can lead to poor nutrient absorption/ utilisation and can inadvertently speed up or slow down your digestion. If it's too fast, then not enough nutrients are absorbed; but if it's too slow, constipation among other problems can result. Balance is key!

The benefits of a healthy digestive system include:
- A healthy immune system
- Healthy hormone regulation
- Elimination of toxins
- Proper stamina and energy generation

IMMUNITY

The digestive system is paramount to the body's immune system. It has been established through research that the higher the quantity and diversity of gut flora, the stronger our immune system is. This means focusing on having a balance of *good* bacteria is essential for defending the body against threats.

70% of our Immune System is part of the Digestive System!

Elevated stress, poor diets, alcohol consumption, antibiotics, illicit drugs all reduce the quantity of good bacteria. The result is an Immune System that is weakened. A weakened immune system leads to the body struggling to fight off invading pathogens.

Your gut health matters more than you can imagine, that's why it's the first topic of discussion.

HORMONE REGULATION

The digestive system plays a significant role in controlling your mood. It does this by producing serotonin in your gastrointestinal (GI) tract. The release of other hormones are also stimulated by the digestive system. These hormones have an impact on how nutrients are absorbed and used in the body.

TOXINS

We feel considerably healthier when our digestive system is healthy, this is because it optimises the elimination of toxins in the body. We excrete these toxins through sweat, urination, bowel movements, mucus secretions, and breathing.
Even though our body regularly uses these methods for toxin elimination, a poor diet can result in the body having problems with identifying and removing toxins. The build up of which causes health complications.

Regular, Consistent bowel movements indicates healthy toxin elimination from the body.

ENERGY & STAMINA

A healthy balanced diet combined with an effectively functioning and fuelled digestive system will generally lead to an increase in energy and stamina. There is a direct correlation between the health of your digestive system and how energy is utilised. This is because the digestive system is responsible for breaking down, absorbing and utilising nutrients that your body uses for energy.
A poorly functioning digestive system will lead to reduced energy, because the cells of the body aren't receiving the nutrients they require through your diet.

BOWEL TRANSIT TIMES

The length of time it takes ingested food to be passed out of the body is known as Bowel Transit Time (BTT).

BTT is an important factor in determining if you are healthy. A healthy BTT results in food working its way through the gastrointestinal tract. During this process harmful toxins are produced and excreted from the body.
Earlier we mentioned that slow digestion is an indicator of poor health. Why? Because if these toxic products move slowly through the gastrointestinal tract, they can and are absorbed into the bloodstream, leading to health complications.

Food Transit Times:

Low fibre diet = 65 - 100 hours
High fibre diet = 20 - 45 hours

Healthy Food Transit Times:

12 - 48 Hours
1 - 2 bowel movements/ day

Mouth ~1 minute
Oesophagus ~4 - 5 seconds
Stomach ~2 - 4 hours
Small intestines ~3 - 5 hours
Colon ~10 hours - A few days

FACTORS IMPACTING BOWEL TRANSIT TIME

The most common factors are listed here in no particular order:

- Behavioural traits
- The liver
- Stress
- Medications
- Climate
- Lifestyle
- Diet
- Age
- Medical conditions
- Hydration

DIGESTIVE HEALTH & THE ROLES OF BACTERIA

Bacteria, also known as 'gut flora' has an important role in both digestion and immunity. Our digestive system contains around 35,000 species of bacteria working symbiotically. They metabolise nutrients and drugs, maintain the structure of the gut's mucosal barrier and protect against invading microorganisms.

If your gut health is poor you could experience a number of diseases:

- Allergies
- Diabetes
- Obesity
- Inflammatory bowel syndrome
- Irritable bowel syndrome

To keep everything you have just read in working order, FIBRE is your best friend!

3-5 servings of Vegetables/ Day
1-2 servings of Fruit/ Day

Depending on your intake, you may benefit from Prebiotic supplements. Ask your Pharmacist/ Chemist for guidance.

FACTORS IMPACTING OUR BODIES RELATED TO THE DIGESTIVE SYSTEM

Note. These are ***possible*** impacts. You may or may not have one, some or all symptoms. Though it is highly unlikely to impossible that you will have all symptoms simultaneously.

FACTOR	SUB-FACTOR	IMPACT
Poor Dietary Choices	Meal Timing	Late meals lead to indigestion, acid reflux, poor sleep. Eating close to exercise, leads to Impaired exercise performance. Poor sleep.
	Meal Composition	Caffeinated drinks, spicy, fatty or large meals reduce quality of sleep
	Eating Style	Eating quickly/ too much leads to bloating, abdominal discomfort/ pain
Poor Hydration		Pebble-like stool, constipation, exhaustion
Inadequate Fibre Intake		Pebble-like stool, cholesterol build up, constipation, reduced gut flora, obesity, gut inflammation, impaired immune system
Smoking & Excessive Alcohol	Smoking	Cancers: Colon, Mouth, Stomach, Oesophagus, Pancreas, Rectal
		Pancreatitis, Gallstones, Gastro-oesophageal reflux disease (GORD - called 'GERD' in the US), Peptic ulcers, Crohn's disease
	Alcohol	Fatty Liver Disease, Cirrhosis (Liver Disease)
		Poor nutrient digestion & absorption
Sedentary Lifestyle		Lack of blood flow to the Digestive system, leads to fat build up around organs. Inefficient transport of nutrients, vitamins and minerals
		Poor waste moveMalest through the digestive system and constipation
		Type 2 Diabetes mellitus, Gastrointestinal & Colorectal cancer, Gallstones
Stress		Decreases Digestive System activity, inflammation and irritation of the gut
Gut Flora Imbalance		Vomiting, dehydration, permanent intestinal damage, cramps
		Abdominal pain, bloating, gas, irregular bowel moveMalests
Genetic	Age	Nutrient deficiencies, physical complications of the gastrointestinal tract
	Gender (WoMales)	Slower gastric emptying, higher risk of developing Irritable Bowel Syndrome, constipation, slower bowel transit times
Ethnicity		Different occurrences of food intolerances, illnesses, and allergies

RECOMMENDED DIETARY INTAKE - FOR A HEALTHY DIGESTIVE SYSTEM

The following (*below*) highlighting 'Recommended Dietary Intakes' (RDI) have been adopted from the Nutrient Reference Values for Australia and New Zealand (NHMRC).

1. Consume 30g of fibre per day
2. Exercise regularly
3. Maintain a healthy weight
4. Reduce smoking and alcohol consumption
5. Incorporate supplements such as (Prebiotics, Probiotics, Zinc & Glutamine)
6. Consume the recommended macronutrient intake for your energy requirements (more detail on this in provided in **Chapters 3, 4 ,5**)
7. Consume whole foods
8. Hydrate adequately (**Chapter 6**)
9. Don't eat 60 minutes before bedtime
10. Take up relaxation activities
11. Chew your food properly, not quickly

CHAPTER 2:

VITAMINS & MINERALS

MICRONUTRIENTS

Your body continuously carries out thousands of chemical reactions at any given moment. Micronutrients, also known as Vitamins and Minerals are compulsory for these reactions to occur. They are responsible for creating Enzymes, Hormones and Other Substances that your body needs for normal growth and development.

Here is a non-exhaustive list of what Vitamins & Minerals ultimately take part in:

- Night vision
- Blood clotting
- Glucose metabolism
- Nerve functioning
- Improved immunity
- Wound healing
- Supports relaxation and constriction of blood vessels
- Regulates fluid volume in the body
- Regulates pH
- Supports normal functioning of cells
- Bone metabolism and strength
- Metabolism of macronutrients

Did you know?

Vitamins are formed from organic matter, e.g. plants and animals

Minerals are formed from inorganic matter, e.g. soil and water

VITAMINS

Consuming a well balanced, varied diet ensures that your body is able to source the correct Vitamins in the required quantities on an uninterrupted, daily basis, failing to do so will lead to deficiencies.

Fact: The body can't make its own Vitamins and Minerals.

If you are unable to derive the micronutrients your body needs from foods because of increased metabolic demands, mal-absorptive issues, or because you do not have access to particular foods (due to budgetary or location reasons), you may need to supplement them into your diet using over the counter vitamin and mineral supplements.

The following Table (*below*) highlighting 'Recommended Dietary Intakes' (RDI) have been adopted from the Nutrient Reference Values for Australia and New Zealand (NHMRC).

RECOMMENDED DIETARY INTAKE - VITAMINS

VITAMIN	RECOMMALESDED DIETARY (DAILY) INTAKE	SOURCES FROM FOOD	BENEFITS
Vitamin A (Retinoids & Carotenoids)	Males: 900 mcg (3,000 IU)	Fortified milk, beef, fish, liver, eggs, mangos, carrots, spinach, pumpkins, squash, sweet potatoes.	Healthy skin, vision, tissue. Supports bone growth.
	WoMales: 700 mcg (2,333 IU)		
Vitamin D	Males/ WoMales:	Oily fish (salmon, tuna, mackerel), cheese, egg yolks, beef liver	Maintenance of healthy levels of calcium and phosphorus in the blood.
	19 - 50yrs - 5 mcg (200IU)		Calcium absorption
	51 - 70yrs - 10 mcg (400IU)		Activates immune system
	71yrs+ - 15 mcg (600 IU)		
Vitamin E	Males: 10 mg	Green leafy vegetables, wheat germ, whole grains, nuts	Neutralises free radicals, protects Vitamin A, lipids from being damaged
	WoMales: 7 mg		
Vitamin K	Males: 70 mcg	Fish, eggs, Brussels sprouts, leafy green vegetables (spinach, kale), broccoli, liver, cauliflower	Blood clotting
	WoMales 60 mcg		Formation of proteins contained in the kidneys, plasma and bones.
			Required for strong bones
Vitamin B1 (Thiamine)	Males: 1.2 mg	Peas, eggs, oats, oranges, nuts & seeds, dried milk, pork, beef, legumes	Helps the body to convert food to energy, healthy skin, hair, muscles and brain function
	WoMales: 1.1 mg		
Vitamin B2 (Riboflavin)	Males:	Almonds, sun-dried tomatoes, lamb, milk, spinach, natural yoghurt	Helps the body to convert food to energy, healthy skin, hair, muscles and brain function
	19 - 70yrs - 1.3 mg		
	>70yrs - 1.6 mg		
	WoMales:		
	19 - 70yrs - 1.1 mg		
	>70yrs - 1.3 mg		
Vitamin B3 (Niacin)	Males: 16 mg	Potatoes, poultry, meat, fish, mushrooms, whole grains	Helps the body to convert food to energy, important for nervous system & brain function. Healthy blood cells and skin
	WoMales: 14 mg		

VITAMIN	RECOMMALESDED DIETARY (DAILY) INTAKE	SOURCES FROM FOOD	BENEFITS
Vitamin B5 (Pantothenic Acid)	Males: 6 mg	Avocados, sunflower seeds, salmon, broccoli, whole grains chicken liver, mushrooms	Helps the body to convert food to energy, aids in the production of fats, neurotransmitters, haemoglobin, and steroid hormones
	WoMales: 4 mg		
Vitamin B6	Males:	Beef liver, fish, non-citrus fruits, potatoes, starchy vegetables, organ meat	Lowers homocysteine levels, aids conversion of neurotransmitter tryptophan into niacin and serotonin, helps produce red blood cells, needed for immune and cognitive function
	19 - 50yrs - 1.3 mg		
	>50yrs: 1.7 mg		
	WoMales:		
	19 - 50yrs - 1.3 mg		
	>50yrs: 1.5 mg		
Vitamin B7 & B8 (Biotin)	Males: 30 mcg	Mushrooms, oats, eggs, kale, calf liver, pork liver	Helps to keep the nervous system, skin, hair, liver and eyes healthy
	WoMales: 25 mcg		
Vitamin B9 (Folic Acid/ Folate)	Males: 400 mcg	Citrus fruits, avocado, asparagus, broccoli, spinarci, collard, Brussels sprouts, turnip greens, nuts, lentils	Synthesis of DNA/ RNA, cell division and growth, healthy red blood production
	WoMales: 400 mcg		
Vitamin B12	Males/ WoMales: 2.4 mcg	Eggs, liver, shellfish, crab, fortified cereals, cheese, red meat, fortified tofu/ soy milk, fish	Healthy nerve cells, production of DNA/ RNA, works with Vit B9 to help make red blood cells, aids iron to function in the body
Vitamin C	Males/ WoMales: 45 mg	Guava, kale, red capsicum, citrus fruits, Brussels sprouts, broccoli, strawberries	Growth & repair of tissue, assists in th production of collagen, healing wounds, repairing and maintaining teeth and bones

MINERALS

Even though they are necessary for your continued functioning, much like Vitamins, your body isn't able to produce Minerals. They are found in soil and water, and must be consumed, albeit in minute quantities. The food you eat, namely plants and animals, contain the Minerals your body needs. How? Plants grow in soil and absorb them. Animals eat plants, animals eat other animals. You eat said plants and animals.
These Minerals must be consumed on an uninterrupted daily basis, otherwise, much like not consuming enough Vitamins, you may end up with a deficiency.

The following Table (*below*) highlighting 'Recommended Dietary Intakes' (RDI) have been adopted from the Nutrient Reference Values for Australia and New Zealand (NHMRC).

RECOMMENDED DIETARY INTAKE - MINERALS

MINERAL	RECOMMALESDED DIETARY (DAILY) INTAKE	SOURCES FROM FOOD	BENEFITS
Iodine	Males/ Females: 150 ug	Salmon, milk, scallops, fish paste, cheese, spinach, green beans, egg yolks	Regulates developMalest, metabolism and growth
Calcium	Males 19 - 70yrs: 1000 mg	Curly parsley, bony fish, boy chow, silverbeet, crab, dairy foods, tahini, almonds	Correct functioning of the cardio vascular system, neuromuscular system and maintenance of all bones
	Males >71yrs: 1300 mg	To increase absorption of Calcium, take with Vitamin D	
	Females 19 -50yrs: 1000 mg		
	Females >51yrs: 1300 mg		
	Male/ Female Maximum: 2500mg		
Chloride	No established values	Lettuce, Celery, Seaweed, olives, rye, tomatoes	Maintains a healthy metabolism
Potassium	Males: 3800 mg	Avocados, seeds, nuts, bananas, cocoa, Vegemite, potatoes, dairy, dried fruits	Maintains blood pressure, transmits electrical pulses, aids in optimal muscle and nerve function, works with sodium as an electrolyte
	Females: 2800 mg		
Magnesium	Males 19 - 30yrs: 400 mg	Almonds, sesame seeds, peanuts, Brazil nuts, dried fruit, yogurt, dark chocolate, sunflower seeds, cocoa	Is required for over 300 biochemical reactions in the body. It is involved in energy production, synthesis of proteins, nerve and muscle function, controlling blood glucose, regulating blood pressure
	Males >31yrs: 225 mg		
	Females 19 -30yrs: 310 mg		
	Females >31yrs: 320 mg		
	Males/ Females Maximum: 350 mg		

MINERAL	RECOMMALESDED DIETARY (DAILY) INTAKE	SOURCES FROM FOOD	BENEFITS
Sulphur	No established values	Lamb, bread, sesame seeds, beefs, sunflower seeds, pork, nuts	Is contained in essential amino acids that are needed for protein synthesis, production of hormones, cells, tissue, antibodies and enzymes
Iron	Males: 8 mg Females 19 - 50yrs: 18 mg Females >50yrs: 8 mg	Dried fruits, leafy green vegetables, seafood, liver, beans, kidneys, red meat	Important part of haemoglobin
	Male/ Female Maximum: 45 mg		
Zinc	Males: 14 mg	Mushrooms, poultry, fish, red meat, legumes, oysters	Healthy function if the immune system, wound healing, cell growth/ division and carbohydrate breakdown
	Females: 8 mg Male/ Female Maximum: 40 mg Males/ Females Maximum: 1100 ug		
Selenium	Males/ Females: 60 ug Male/ Female Maximum: 400 ug	Mushrooms, fish, brain nuts, sesame seeds, oysters, eggs yolks	Prevents free radical damage
Copper	Males: 1.7 mg Female: 1.2 mg Male/ Female Maximum: 10 mg	Dried fruits, Brazil nuts, dark chocolate, lobster, lamb liver, sunflower seeds	Forms a part of enzymes, helps to metabolise iron
Chloride	No established values	Lettuce, Celery, Seaweed, olives, rye, tomatoes	Maintains a healthy metabolism
Sodium	Males/ Females: 460 - 920 mg Male/Female Maximum: 2300 mg	Canned fish, bread, feta cheese, stock cubes, table salt, anchovies	Important electrolyte, maintains fluid balance, essential for enzyme function, and muscle contractions
Manganese	Males: 5.5 mg	Hazelnuts, tofu, whole grains, macadamia nuts	Needed for bone formation and structure, important for metabolism
Fluoride	Females: 5 mg Males: 4 mg Females: 3 mg	Lettuce, fish, water, duck, liquorice, fish paste, avocado	Strong teeth, enamel, and reduced decay of teeth

MINERAL	RECOMMALESDED DIETARY (DAILY) INTAKE	SOURCES FROM FOOD	BENEFITS
	Male/ Female Maximum: 10 mg		
Chromium	Males: 35 mg	Sultanas, olives, curly parsley, red wine, cheddar cheese, bread, spinach. Cottage cheese	Regulates blood sugar, aids in glucose transport, and the metabolism of protein and fats
	Females: 25 mg		
Molybdenum	Males/ Females: 45 ug	Cparsley, almondsoconut, peanut butter, cream, lamb liver, cheddar cheese, curly	Enzyme catalyst, helps the breakdown of amino acids
	Male/ Female Maximum: 2000 ug		

CHAPTER 3:

PROTEIN

WHAT IS PROTEIN? WHY IS IT IMPORTANT?

Protein is a macronutrient that contains nitrogen, and is formed from amino acids. As the building blocks of protein, amino acids are sometimes referred to as the building blocks of life. Organisms consist of thousands of proteins. They define what it is, how it looks and even how it behaves.

It cannot be understated that Protein is an essential nutrient and is quite literally involved in EVERY biochemical process that takes place in your body. A diet that does not contain enough protein will lead to fatigue, weakness, slowed recovery from exercise, muscle deterioration and poor health outcomes overall. Protein is also an energy containing macronutrient yielding 17kJ (4 Calories) per gram.

Some of the processes that protein is involved in include:

- Immune function
- Healthy nails, hair and skin
- Tissue repair
- Energy production
- Hormone production
- Enzyme production

SOURCES OF PROTEIN

It is very important to note that foods that are regarded as containing protein, do not contain 100% protein, for example 100g of beef, DOES NOT contain 100g of protein. Beef is a *source* of protein. The amount of protein is linked to the bioavailability of the protein in the source. Bioavailability simply refers to how well your body can and will use the protein from the source that you consumed.

The following Table (*below*) highlighting 'Sources of Protein' have been adopted from the United States Department of Agriculture, 'Nutritive Value of Foods' Guide.

FOOD	**PROTEIN PER 100 GRAMS**
Lamb	
Boneless Lamb leg	28g
Lamb Cutlets	28g
Lamb Chops (with bone)	32g
Lamb backstrap	24g
Beef	
Lean Beef mince	28g
Lean sirloin steak	30g
Lean tenderloin steak	28g
Seafood	
Salmon (Poached)	25g
Tuna	27g
Snapper (Baked)	26g
Prawns/ Shrimp	24g
Cod	18g
Lobster	20g
Scallops	24g

FOOD	PROTEIN PER 100 GRAMS
Squid	18g
Crab	19g
Mussels	24g
Clams	26g
Octopus	30g
Eel	18g
Haddock (Fish)	18g
Oysters	9g
Caviar	25g
Pork	
Lean tenderloin (Pan fried)	28g
Bacon (Canadian style - fried)	24g
Poultry	
Chicken breast (Roasted /Skin off)	30g
Chicken thigh (Roasted/ Skin off)	26g
Duck	19g
Turkey	29g
Eggs	
Eggs (whole) x2	12g
Eggs (Whites)	11g
Duck eggs	13g
Legumes & Grains	
Chickpeas (Cooked)	19g
Tahini	22g
Lentils (Cooked)	10g
Brown rice (Steamed)	3g
White rice (Basmati/ Steamed)	3g
Kidney beans (raw)	24g
Soybeans (Cooked	17g
Baked Beans	6g
Oats	17g
Edamame	13g
Quinoa	4g
Nuts & Seeds	
Walnuts	16g
Chia seeds	15g
Flexseeds	19g
Peanuts	26g
Almonds	21g
Sunflower seeds	21g
Pumpkin seeds	19g
Pistachio nuts	21g

FOOD	PROTEIN PER 100 GRAMS
Cashew nuts	18g
Macadamia nuts	11g
Peanut butter	25g
Pecan nuts	9g
Dairy	
Low fat Milk	9g
Full cream Milk	8g
Cheese	25g
Cottage cheese	11g
Low fat Greek yoghurt	10g
Non-dairy Milk	
Soy milk	3.3g
Almond milk (unsweetened)	1.6g
Oat milk	1g
Supplements	
Whey protein isolate (WPI)	92g
Whey protein concentrate (WPC)	80g
Pea protein	75g
Brown rice protein	77g
Soy protein	80g
Other	
Tofu	18g
Coconut yoghurt	2g
Coconut milk	2g
Peas	5g

HOW TO CALCULATE HOW MUCH PROTEIN IS IN A PORTION OF FOOD

This example will use a 156g Sirloin steak.

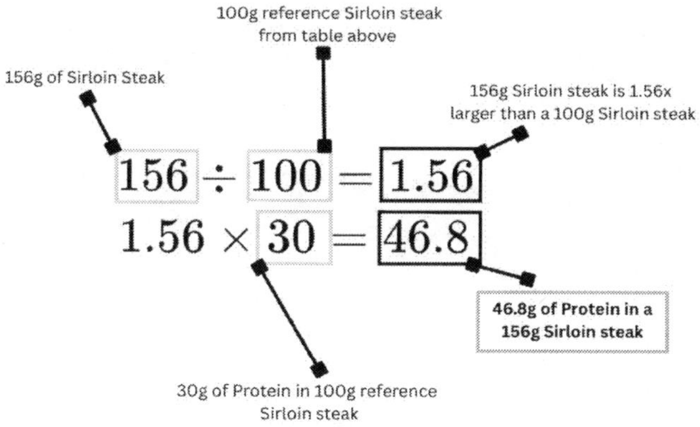

RECOMMENDED DIETARY INTAKE - PROTEIN

The amount of protein you need will depend on how active you are during the day. Even if you sit all day without any exertion, your body still needs protein for its biochemical processes, as mentioned earlier. If you are sedentary (sit more often than not) pay attention to the moderate part of the range below. If you are an older adult, pay attention to the higher end of the range.

The following Table (*below*) highlighting 'Recommended Dietary Intakes' (RDI) have been adopted from the Nutrient Reference Values for Australia and New Zealand (NHMRC).

ACTIVITY LEVEL	RDI
Sedentary (Sit down job, no physical activity)	Females - 0.75g - 1.0g of protein per kilogram of body weight per day
	Males - 0.84 - 1.0g of protein per kilogram of body weight per day
Light Activity (1 - 2 days light physical activity/ week)	0.75 - 1.2g of protein per kilogram of body weight per day
Moderate Intensity Activity (2 - 4 days moderate - intense activity/ week	1.2 - 1.5g of protein per kilogram of body weight per day
High Intensity Activity (4+ days high intensity activity/ week)	1.5 - 2.0g of protein per kilogram of body weight per day

CHAPTER 4:

CARBOHYDRATES & FIBRE

WHAT ARE CARBOHYDRATES?

Organic compounds that are made up of starches and sugars are known as Carbohydrates. They are part of the Macronutrient family, and are considered to be an immediate and major energy source for not only the human body, but for most other organisms as well. When the body metabolises carbohydrates, they break them down into simple sugars, such as glucose, galactose (found in dairy products), and fructose (found in fruit).
The contents of carbohydrates play an important role in how sugar from their metabolism is released into our bloodstreams, the quality and quantity of our gut flora, the regulation of our bowel movements, and the how full we feel. These benefits are gained from macronutrients because they contain varying levels of fibre and starch. The body is able to break starch down into the simple sugars mentioned earlier, but fibres are not digested at all and simply pass through to excretion. It is the action of fibre that leads to the quality and quantity of our gut flora, the regulation of our bowel movements, and the how full we feel.
Carbohydrates are also an energy containing macronutrient yielding 17kJ (4 Calories) per gram.

WHY IS IT IMPORTANT?

There are three important roles that Carbohydrates play in our bodies:

- Provides our bodies with energy
- Provides our bodies with immediate energy
- Helps keep our digestive system healthy (as discussed in **Chapter 1**)

SOURCES OF CARBOHYDRATES

It is very important to note that foods that are regarded as containing carbohydrates do not contain 100% carbohydrates, for example 100g of brown rice, DOES NOT contain 100g of carbohydrates. Brown rice is a *source* of carbohydrates. The amount of nutrients (carbohydrates) present in foods is linked to the type of carbohydrate (e.g. type of rice or the variety of banana), how it is stored and cooked.

The following Table (*below*) highlighting 'Sources of Carbohydrates' have been adopted from the United States Department of Agriculture, 'Nutritive Value of Foods' Guide.

FOOD	CARBOHYDRATES PER 100 GRAMS
Milk Chocolate	57g
Hot dog bun	57g
Hamburger bun	50g
Tortilla	46g
Plain chips (Crisps)	46g
White bread	46g
Wholemeal bread	38g
Cassava	38g
Jasmine Rice	32g
Basmati rice	31g
White pasta	31g
Long grain rice	28g
Taro	27g
Australian meat pie (pastry)	24g
Banana (white fruit part only)	23g

FOOD	CARBOHYDRATES PER 100 GRAMS
Brown rice	23g
Potato	21g
Sweet potato	20g
Taco	20g
Lentils	20g
Apple	14g
Pineapple	13g
Mandarin	13g
Orange	12g
Apricots	11g
Strawberries	8g
Watermelon	8g
Low-fat Greek yoghurt	6g
Full-fat Greek yoghurt	5g
Full cream milk	4.7g
Beer	4g

HOW TO CALCULATE HOW MUCH CARBOHYDRATES ARE IN A PORTION OF FOOD

This example will use 165g of White pasta.

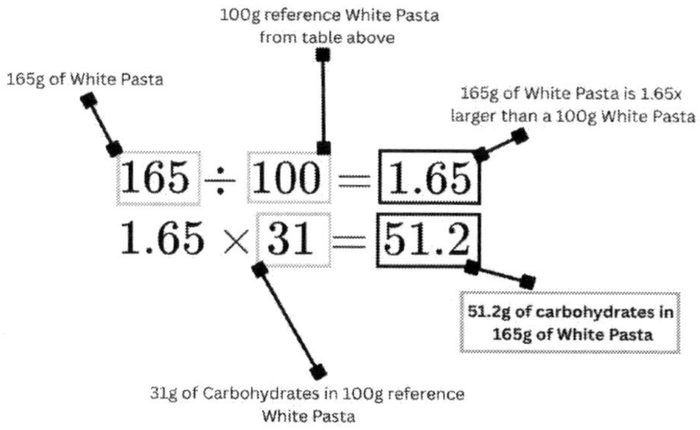

RECOMMENDED DIETARY INTAKE - CARBOHYDRATES

If you are using an app such as 'MyFitnessPal', 'Chronometer', 'LoseIt', 'LifeSum' or similar, ensure that the percentage of energy from Carbohydrates in the app meets the requirements of the table below. If you consume too much carbohydrates with a weight loss goal, you will not lose weight. If you consume too few carbohydrates you will experience poor mental health outcomes and significantly reduced energy for day-to-day activities. Balance is key.

The following Table (*below*) highlighting 'Recommended Dietary Intakes' (RDI) have been adopted from the Nutrient Reference Values for Australia and New Zealand (NHMRC).

ACTIVITY LEVEL	RDI	IMPORTANT NOTE
Sedentary (Sit down job, no physical activity)	20 - 30% of energy intake	Ensure adequate fats and protein for energy
Light Activity (1 - 2 days light physical activity/ week)	30 - 35% of energy intake	Ensure adequate fats and protein for energy
Moderate Intensity Activity (2 - 4 days moderate - intense activity/ week)	40 - 50% of energy intake	
High Intensity Activity (4+ days high intensity activity/ week)	60%+ of energy intake	

FIBRE

Dietary fibre refers to parts of fruits, vegetables, legumes and beans that are edible, but cannot be digested or absorbed by the body. They can however partially or completely ferment in the large intestines.
Fibre is an important factor in how your body controls (decreases) cholesterol levels, regulates your blood sugar levels, gives you a feeling of fullness after eating, and makes bowel movements easier.

RECOMMENDED DIETARY INTAKE - FIBRE

The following Table (*below*) highlighting 'Recommended Dietary Intakes' (RDI) have been adopted from the Nutrient Reference Values for Australia and New Zealand (NHMRC).

AGE (YEARS)	DAILY INTAKE (ADEQUATE INTAKE)
Males 19yrs+	30g
Females 19yrs+	25g

CHAPTER 5:

DIETARY FATS

WHAT ARE DIETARY FATS?

Dietary fats are the last essential member of the Macronutrient family along side Proteins and Carbohydrates. These nutrients are essential to the functioning of the human body. Yes! Your body needs fats to survive. There is no such thing as a zero fat diet, attempting to lead a diet free of fats will lead to medical complications, often serious.

Dietary fats are also an energy containing macronutrient yielding 37kJ (9 Calories) per gram.

WHY ARE THEY IMPORTANT?

Dietary fats play an important role in the following processes in the human body, they are manipulated by the body to create fatty acids that are in turn used to create essential fats:

- Important part of cell walls (**Phospholipids**)
- Building of required fats from other fats (**Free fatty acids**)
- Important part of hormone production, cell walls, and fat-soluble vitamins (**Cholesterol**)
- Fat storage in adipose tissue (**Triglycerides**)
- Fats plays an important role in the following:
    - Maintaining healthy cholesterol levels in the body
    - Reducing cardiovascular risk
    - Blood vessel elasticity
    - Maintaining healthy skin, hair and strong nails
    - Normal nerve function
    - Blood clots
    - Storing some vitamins
    - Improving brain development and functioning
    - Increasing immunity and decreasing inflammation
    - Decreasing your risk of developing anxiety and depression
    - Regulating hunger

Note: "Plays an important role in" means that the process CANNOT complete without it.

Please refer to the section in this chapter labelled 'Recommended Dietary Intake - Dietary Fats' to learn how much Dietary Fats you should consume. The information provided above is in no way an advocation to increase your dietary fat consumption to unhealthy levels. Consuming too much dietary fats leads to health complications. Again, balance is key.

TYPES OF DIETARY FATS

There are four main types of fats:

- Trans fats
- Saturated fats
- Monounsaturated fats (Unsaturated Fat)
- Polyunsaturated fats (Unsaturated Fat)

TRANS FATS

Trans fats are derived from two sources, namely animals (deer, cows, goats and sheep), and industrial processing of food. Naturally occurring trans fats from animals are found in small quantities, however the existence of trans fat in our diets primary comes from Western diets that contain foods and oils that have been processed.

Products that contain trans fats include:

- Cakes, biscuits and other processed baked products
- Hydrogenated margarines (solidified vegetable fats)

- Pizza, pies, hot dogs and other processed meet products
- Hot chips, fish and other deep fried products

Trans fats increase cholesterol known as LDL-cholesterol in your bloodstream, while reducing HDL-cholesterol (beneficial cholesterol). LDL-cholesterol is a major risk factor in heart disease.
It is important to note that reducing Trans fats in your diet should be a priority. The World Health Organisation recommends that Trans fats only make up 1% of your diet.

SATURATED FATS

Saturated fats can be consumed from healthy and unhealthy food sources. Healthy sources include some meats, eggs and dairy. Products such as Kefir and yogurt contain beneficial probiotics that are essential for gut microbiota.
But, much like Trans Fats these foods are sources of unhealthy saturated fats:

- Processed foods such as hot chips, fish and other deep fried products
- Hot dogs, pizza, pies and other processed meet products
- Cakes, biscuits and other processed baked products

Animal and plant based products that contain saturated fats include:

- Coconut milk, coconut cream and coconut oil
- Lard, tallow and ghee
- Milk, yoghurt and cheese

UNSATURATED FATS

Unsaturated fats are dietary fats you should consume more often. These are healthy 'good' fats. There are two types, Monounsaturated and Polyunsaturated. Unsaturated fats reduce the build up on cholesterol in your arteries, which in turn decreases your risk of strokes and heart disease.

Unsaturated fats play important roles in the body, these include:

- Reducing and improving inflammation
- Maintaining body weight
- Reducing blood pressure for patients diagnosed with hypertension
- Improving the function of your blood vessels
- Stabilising your heart rhythm
- Reduce the amount of triglycerides, a fat known to harden arteries
- Building strong cell membranes
- Helping patients with type II diabetes

MONOUNSATURATED FATS

HDL Cholesterol - High-density lipoprotein (Considered to be 'good' cholesterol because it is able to absorb LDL-cholesterol and transport it to your liver where it is discarded by the body)

LDL Cholesterol - Low-density lipoprotein (Considered to be 'bad' cholesterol because it can build up as plaque in your arteries)

Monounsaturated fats have some benefits including:

- Reducing your cardiovascular risk (the have an impact on HDL & LDL cholesterol levels)
- Can reduce inflammation

SOURCES OF MONOUNSATURATED FATS

Monounsaturated fats are found in animal and plant based foods. The table below lists sources of food that are high in Monounsaturated fats (the 'Good' fat).

The following Table (*below*) highlighting 'Sources of Monounsaturated Fats' have been adopted from the United States Department of Agriculture, 'Nutritive Value of Foods' Guide.

FOOD	MONOUNSATURATED FATS PER 100 GRAMS
Eggs	4g
Pumpkin seeds	6g
Pork	6g
Avocados	10g
Olives	15g
Sunflower seeds	15g
Cashew nuts	24g
Peanuts	24g
Pistachio nuts	25g
Almonds	31g
Olive Oil	555 - 83g

POLYUNSATURATED FATS

Polyunsaturated fats are generally found in food sourced from plants, oily fish and some oils. It is important to maintain a diet that contains polyunsaturated fats as the body benefits from this type of fat. These benefits include:

- A decreased risk of developing heart disease
- A decreased risk of developing type II diabetes
- Regulation of blood cholesterol levels

Polyunsaturated fats are classified into two groups:

- Omega-3 fatty acids - these include Eicosapentaenoic acid (EPA), Docosahexaenoic acid (DHA) & Alpha-linolenic acid (ALA)
- Omega-6 fatty acids - these include linolenic acids and others

Your body isn't able to create Omega 3 & 6 fatty acids from other fatty acids as mentioned earlier, as such it is essential that you consume them from your diet.

OMEGA-3 FATTY ACIDS

Omega-3 fatty acids have numerous benefits and play crucial roles in our bodies, these include:

- Health of your heart
- Joint health
- Brain health
- Maintaining your vision
- Reducing inflammation n your body
- Conserving testosterone levels
- Insulin sensitivity
- Protein synthesis
- Increasing growth hormone levels

SOURCES OF OMEGA-3 FATTY ACIDS

The following Table (*below*) highlighting 'Sources of Omega-3 Fatty Acids' have been adopted from the United States Department of Agriculture, 'Nutritive Value of Foods' Guide.

FOODS CONTAINING OMEGA-3 FATTY ACIDS
Garlic
Walnuts
Oily fish (mackerel, salmon, sardines)
Sesame seeds, flaxseeds
Whole eggs
Spinach, collards, kale
Olive oil
Avocados

OMEGA-6 FATTY ACIDS

Omega-6 fatty acids have numerous benefits and play crucial roles in our bodies, these include:

- Production of cell membranes
- Cell signalling
- Blood vessel dilation
- Preventing blood clots
- Reducing inflammation
- Treating arthritis, high blood pressure, and eczema

SOURCES OF OMEGA-6 FATTY ACIDS

The following Table (*below*) highlighting 'Sources of Omega-6 Fatty Acids' have been adopted from the United States Department of Agriculture, 'Nutritive Value of Foods' Guide.

FOODS CONTAINING OMEGA-6 FATTY ACIDS
Eggs
Evening primrose oil
Deep fried foods
Butter, cheese, milk and cream
Pistachio nuts and sunflower seeds
Olive oil and olives
Sunflower oil, soybean oil and canola oil
Baked goods (Commercial products)

RECOMMENDED DIETARY INTAKE - DIETARY FATS

The following Table (*below*) highlighting 'Recommended Dietary Intakes' (RDI) have been adopted from the Nutrient Reference Values for Australia and New Zealand (NHMRC).

TYPE OF DIETARY FAT	RDI
Trans fats	<1% of total energy consumption
Monounsaturated Fats	50-65% of total dietary fat consumption
Polyunsaturated Fat Omega-3	250 - 500 mg per day
Polyunsaturated Fat Combined ALA-3, DHA, EPA	1g per day
Polyunsaturated Fat Omega-6	4 - 10% of total energy consumption

CHAPTER 6:

HYDRATION

WHAT IS HYDRATION?

You will have heard that our bodies are made up of two thirds water in relation to our body weight. It is therefore very important that you consume water constantly throughout the day in order to maintain the healthy functioning of your body.

A great way to check your level of hydration is by observing the colour of your urine. The following colours are important:

- Clear - you may have over hydrated
- Pale yellow - you are well hydrated
- Dark yellow - you are dehydrated

THE ROLE OF WATER?

Water is involved in many processes throughout your body, these include:

- It helps when you swallow
- It lubricates your cells
- It regulates you body temperature
- It helps eliminates waste
- Water is the medium in which many of the chemical reactions in your body occur

DEHYDRATION

The amount of water your body needs is individualised. There are many factors that control your fluid requirements and these include things such as the climate you live or work in, your age, the type of work you do, your weight and any other physical activity that you take part in.
If you live in a hot and/ or humid climate your fluid requirements will be significantly higher than someone living in a cooler climate, or those that are older and or live a sedentary lifestyle. We lose water through sweat. Sweat (largely water) regulates our skin temperature. Water regulates our body temperature internally.
A drop of as little as 2% of your body water will cause symptoms of dehydration.

You will notice these symptoms if you are dehydrated, or are getting close to it:

- Nausea
- Elevated body temperature
- Elevated heart rate
- Excessive thirst
- Lethargy
- Headaches
- Reduce blood pressure
- A reduction in your ability to concentration
- A reduction in cognitive function

ELECTROLYTES

Two electrolytes are imperative for hydration, Sodium and Potassium. These electrolytes work together to maintain your blood pressure and balance the water within your body. Without adequate intake of these minerals you will experience dehydration, as well as mental apathy, loss of your appetite, muscle cramps, diarrhoea, sweating, and excessive vomiting among other symptoms.

RECOMMENDED DIETARY INTAKE - ELECTROLYTES

The following Table (*below*) highlighting 'Recommended Dietary Intakes' (RDI) have been adopted from the Nutrient Reference Values for Australia and New Zealand (NHMRC).

ELECTROLYTE	RDI
Sodium	Males/ Females: 460 - 920 mg
	Male/Female Maximum: 2300 mg
Potassium	Males: 3800 mg
	Females: 2800 mg

RECOMMENDED DIETARY INTAKE - WATER

This recommendation DOES NOT take into account extra activity such as exercise. Please use the table below as a guide. If you are living or working in hotter/ humid climates, your fluid intake will need to be higher. Refer to the urine colour guide above. Experiment with different quantities of water consumption until your urine is regularly pale yellow in colour.
Please do not consume excessive amounts of water in one go as it can cause your cells to rupture.

Drink one glass every 15 minutes if you are feeling dehydrated. Seek out electrolyte sources. Seek out medical attention as soon as possible for severe symptoms.

The following Table (*below*) highlighting 'Recommended Dietary Intakes' (RDI) have been adopted from the Nutrient Reference Values for Australia and New Zealand (NHMRC).

GENDER	RDI
Male/ Female	30 - 35mL per kilogram of body weight per day

CHAPTER 7:

ALCOHOL

NON-ESSENTIAL MACRONUTRIENT - ALCOHOL

It may surprise you to know that Alcohol is considered a Macronutrient, though unlike Protein, Carbohydrates and Dietary Fats, it is not an essential Macronutrient. Alcohol is not needed by the human body for any processes, and therefore is unnecessary for your health and wellbeing or survival.

ENERGY FROM ALCOHOL

Alcohol, though not an essential macronutrient, Alcohol is considered to be part of the macronutrient family because it yields energy. One gram of alcohol provides the body with 29kJ of energy or approximately 7 Calories per gram. In comparison, Dietary fats contain 38kJ of energy and 9 Calories per gram. Because of the excessive amount of energy found in alcohol and the fact that it contains no vitamins or minerals, it is regarded as 'empty Calories'.

The following Table (*below*) highlighting 'Recommended Dietary Intakes' (RDI) have been adopted from the Nutrient Reference Values for Australia and New Zealand (NHMRC).

TYPE OF ALCOHOLIC DRINK	ENERGY (KJ)	CALORIES (KCAL)
150mL Red wine (13% Alc. Vol)	490kJ	117 cal
150mL White wine (11.5% Alc. Vol)	440kJ	105 cal
150mL Reduced alcohol red wine (8 - 9% Alc. Vol)	340kJ	81 cal
150mL Reduced alcohol white wine (8 - 9% Alc. Vol)	320kJ	76 cal
150mL Champagne (12% Alc. Vol)	420kJ	100 cal
30mL Shot of spirits + 170mL of soft drink (40% Alc. Vol)	520kJ	124 cal
1x Bottle full strength beer (4.8% Alc. Vol)	570kJ	136 cal
1x Bottle light beer (2.7% Alc. Vol)	400kJ	96 cal

ALCOHOL CONSUMPTION - THINGS TO KNOW

It is important that you moderate your alcohol consumption as part of a healthy diet. There is some evidence that suggests that drinking red wine can have some benefits when consumed as part of a healthy diet, but it is often the case that not drinking alcohol at all is better for your health outcomes.
There are several impacts that the energy from alcohol can have on your long-term health outcomes. If it is your intention to become healthier, and to achieve the health goals listed below, moderating your consumption of alcohol can be a great assistance in reaching your goal.

- Improve your energy levels
- Improve your relationship with family, friends, workmates and significant others
- Lose weight (if this is your goal)
- Regulate your blood sugar
- Reduce binge drinking
- Reduce your risk of developing diseases such as heart and/ or liver disease and cancer

HOW TO REDUCE YOUR ALCOHOL INTAKE

There are several different ways to reduce your alcohol intake. These include some or all of the following depending on your goals and circumstances.

- Don't keep alcohol in your home
- Buy smaller quantities of alcohol (as an example, purchase a 6 pack rather than a case/ carton)
- Drink low or mid-strength beer instead of full strength varieties
- Drink only during social occasions
- Drink one glass of wine, instead of two/ three, a bottle
- When using mixers, choose low Calorie options like soda water

GUIDE TO STANDARD DRINKS

The following Table (*below*) highlighting 'Guide to Standard Guide' have been adopted from the Department of Health and Aged Care, Australian Government, Stand Drinks Guide.

TYPE OF DRINK	QUANTITY (ML)/ STRENGTH	ALCOHOL QUANTITY (ALC. VOL)	NUMBER OF STANDARD DRINKS
Beer (Served in a glass)	Full strength - 285mL	4.8%	1.1
	Mid strength - 285mL	3.5%	0.8
	Low strength - 285mL	2.7%	0.6
	Full strength - 425mL	4.8%	1.6
	Mid strength - 425mL	3.5%	1.2
	Low strength - 425mL	2.7%	0.9
Beer (Bottles/ Cans)	Full strength - 375mL	4.8%	1.4
	Mid strength - 375mL	3.5%	1.0
	Low strength - 375mL	2.7%	0.8
Case of beer (24 pack)	Full strength - 375mL	4.8%	34
	Mid strength - 375mL	3.5%	24
	Low strength - 375mL	2.7%	19
Wine (Red & Port)	150mL - Restaurant serving size	13.5%	1.6
	100mL	13.5%	1.0
	750mL - bottle	13.5%	8
	Cask of red wine 4L	13.5%	43
	Cask of red wine 2L	13.5%	21
	60mL - Port	17.5%	0.9
	Cask of Port	17.5%	28
White wine	150mL - Restaurant serving size	11.5%	1.4
	100mL	11.5%	0.9
	Cask of white wine 4L	11.5%	36
	Cask of white wine 2L	11.5%	18
Champagne	150mL - Restaurant serving size	12%	1.4
	750mL bottle	12%	7.1
Spirits	30mL	40%	1.0
	700mL bottle	40%	22

TYPE OF DRINK	QUANTITY (ML)/ STRENGTH	ALCOHOL QUANTITY (ALC. VOL)	NUMBER OF STANDARD DRINKS
Ready to drink Spirits	275mL	5%	1.1
	330mL	5%	1.2
	660mL	5%	2.6
	275mL	7%	1.5
	330mL	7%	1.8
	660mL	7%	3.6
Pre-mixed Spirits	250mL	5%	1.0
	300mL	5%	1.2
	375mL	5%	1.5
	440mL	5%	1.7
	250mL	7 - 10%	1.4 - 1.9
	300mL	7%	1.6
	375mL	7%	2.1
	440mL	7%	2.4

RECOMMENDED DIETARY INTAKE - ALCOHOL

The recommended dietary intake for Alcohol is *zero*.

But...

Drinking alcohol is a personal choice, and making informed decisions is important.

The National Health and Medical Research Council (NHMRC) recommends that adults consume:

No more than **Two Standard Drinks** per day over any given week, and **No more than Four Standard** drinks in one session.

CHAPTER 8:

DISCRETIONARY ITEMS

WHAT ARE DISCRETIONARY ITEMS, AND WHY AREN'T THEY IMPORTANT?

You know Discretionary items by their common term, 'Junk Food'. These are foods and drinks that are not required by the human body for any processes, and therefore is unnecessary for your health and wellbeing or survival. Examples include:

- Alcohol
- Packet chips
- Pies
- Hot chips
- Juice
- Soft drinks
- Pastries
- Cakes
- Sweets
- Lollies
- Chocolates
- Other confectionary

Discretionary items are energy dense, they do not contain fibre or the nutrients that are found in fresh whole foods such as fruits, vegetables and nuts. These items are very likely to contain Trans fats. As we found out earlier, Trans fats increase cholesterol known as LDL-cholesterol in your bloodstream, while reducing HDL-cholesterol (beneficial cholesterol). LDL-cholesterol is a major risk factor in heart disease.

It is important to note that reducing Trans fats in your diet should be a priority. The World Health Organisation recommends that Trans fats only make up 1% of your diet. Unfortunately, given that all of the items listed above contain trans fats, it is very likely that you are consuming considerably over this amount, thus increasing your risk of heart disease.

BREAKING DOWN DISCRETIONARY ITEMS BY CONTENT

The following Table (*below*) highlighting 'Discretionary items by content' have been adopted from the Nutrient Reference Values for Australia and New Zealand (NHMRC).

HIGH IN ALCOHOL	HIGH IN TRANS FATS	HIGH IN REFINED SUGAR	HIGH IN TRANS FATS & REFINED SUGAR
Port	Chips	Fuirt juice	Muesli bars
Liqueur Sherry	Commercial pies Commercial pizzas	Soft drinks Tomato sauce (ketchups), BBQ sauce	Chocolates Cakes
Spirits	Processed meats	Coconut sugar, maple syrup, honey, agave syrup	Biscuits
Wine Beer	Some dressing / sauces Deep fried foods	Confectionary Marmalades and jams	Ice cream Doughnuts
Mixed alcoholic drinks	Corn products (chips, enchiladas, tacos, nachos	Energy drinks	Muffins

AMOUNT OF SUGAR FOUND IN COMMON FOODS

The following Table (*below*) highlighting 'The amount of sugar in common foods' have been adopted from the Nutrient Reference Values for Australia and New Zealand (NHMRC).

FOOD	SUGAR (GRAMS)	TEASPOONS (TSP) OF SUGAR PER SERVE	PERCENTAGE OF SUGAR
360mL Coke	38g	10 tsp	11%
1x Chocolate chip muffin	30g	7.5g	29%
120g ice cream	28g	7 tsp	21%
250mL fruit juice	23g	6 tsp	9%
1x Chocolate donut	18g	4.5 tsp	27%
1 tablespoon honey	17g	2.5 tsp	82%
1 tablespoon jam	10g	2.5 tsp	49%
2x Shortbread biscuits	9.5g	5 tsp	28%
30mL tomato sauce	8g	2 tsp	26%
1x Chewy muesli bar	6g	1.5	17%

RECOMMENDED DIETARY INTAKE - DISCRETIONARY ITEMS

A serving of discretionary items is equivalent to 600kJ (150 Calories).

The following Table (*below*) highlighting 'Recommended Dietary Intakes' (RDI) have been adopted from the Nutrient Reference Values for Australia and New Zealand (NHMRC).

ASSOCIATION	MALES	FEMALES
Australian Dietary Guidelines	Reduce how often the foods are consumed and the quantity when consumed.	
World Health Organisation	<10% of your total daily energy should be derived from sugars	
American Heart Association	<9 teaspoons of sugar per day	<6 teaspoons of sugar per day

CHAPTER 9:

ENERGY

WHAT IS ENERGY?

It may sound like a silly question, but if you don't understand how much you need and how much is actually in the foods you eat, obesity may be in your future. Earlier chapters have covered how much you need through 'Recommended Dietary Intake' sections, so here we will focus on energy itself.
Your body uses energy to laugh, for your heart to beat, to breathe and for exercise (and EVERYTHING else). You will have come across the two units that energy is measured in, Calories (Cal) and Kilojoules (kJ). 4.186kJ is equivalent to 1 Calorie.

THE AMOUNT OF ENERGY IN EACH MACRONUTRIENT

The following Table (*below*) highlighting 'Recommended Dietary Intakes' (RDI) have been adopted from the Nutrient Reference Values for Australia and New Zealand (NHMRC).

ENERGY SOURCE (PER GRAM)	KILOJOULES (KJ)	CALORIES (KCAL)
Fats	37.7kJ	9
Alcohol	29.3kJ	7
Carbohydrates	16.7kJ	4
Protein	16.7kJ	4

ENERGY BALANCE

When you consume enough energy to meet your energy needs for the day, this is called energy balance. If you consume more than the energy that you need for the day, you will put on weight. Similarly, if you consume less energy than you need for the day, you will lose weight.
It is very important to note that if your goal is weight gain or loss, you should adopt a 'food as an energy source' mentality. We tend to eat whatever we *feel* like and don't really concern ourselves with nutrition. But when adopting one of these goals, it becomes the reason for your success or failure.

We'll go over Basic Metabolic Rate (BMR) and Estimated Energy Requirement (EER) soon, but it is important for you to know that the amount of energy from food that you need depends on things like your level of physical activity, your age, gender, height, and weight.

BASE METABOLIC RATE (BMR)?

Base metabolic rate refers to your individual energy requirement during rest. It is often used interchangeably with Resting Metabolic Rate (RMR), even though there is a difference between the two. BMR is far more accurate as it takes into account your activity level, age, body composition and weight. RMR doesn't use all of the metrics that BMR uses, and so it isn't relied upon for accurate information. BMR & RMR measure the energy required for Blood circulation, Breathing and Thermoregulation (body temperature regulation).
If you are unwell or injured your BMR can be much higher as the body will demand more energy to heal and fight disease. You will note shortly that BMR is the largest energy expenditure when we run through how to calculate your Estimated Energy Requirements.

Metabolic rate has two parts:

- Basal Metabolic Rate (BMR)
- Total Daily Energy Expenditure (TDEE)

ESTIMATED ENERGY REQUIREMENTS (EER)

Estimated Energy Requirements is the amount of energy your body needs to maintain a healthy energy balance. This takes into account your activity level, height, weight , gender and age. The Harris-Benedict formula is a widely used method for determining your BMR.

To calculate your BMR, use the Harris-Benedict formula that is relevant for your gender. Males generally have a higher lean body weight percentage than Females. It is lean body weight that increases your BMR.

The Harris-Benedict formula is presented below:

Males $$BMR = 66.44 + (13.75 \times W) + (5.0 \times H) - (6.77 \times A)$$

Females $$BMR = 655.1 + (9.56 \times W) + (1.85 \times H) - (4.68 \times A)$$

W - Weight (kg); **H** - Height (cm); **A** - Age (yrs)

PHYSICAL ACTIVITY LEVEL (PAL)

In order to calculate your total Estimated Energy Requirements (EER) you must now multiply your BMR by a Physical Activity Level (PAL) activity factor from the table below:

ACTIVITY LEVEL	ACTIVITY FACTOR	ACTIVITY DESCRIPTION	ACTIVE PERIOD
Very Sedentary	1.2	Bed/ Chair, smaller frame body, no activity	None
Sedentary	1.3 - 1.4	Sit down job, no physical activity	Light leisure activities
Light Activity	1.5 - 1.6	2 - 3 days light physical activity/ week	30 - 60 minutes of exercise
Moderate Intensity Activity	1.6 - 1.8	3 - 4 days moderate - intense activity/ week	45 - 60 minutes exercise
High Intensity Activity	1.8	4+ days high intensity activity/ week	4 - 5 hours of physical exertion, includes laborious work

EXAMPLE 'EER' CALCULATION USING 'BMR' & 'PAL'

$$BMR = 66.44 + (13.75 \times W) + (5.0 \times H) - (6.77 \times A)$$
$$BMR = 66.44 + (13.75 \times 104) + (5.0 \times 189) - (6.77 \times 32)$$ → Multiply out each bracket first, then add/ subtract
$$BMR = 66.44 + (1430) + (945) - (216.64)$$
$$BMR = 2224.8$$

$$PAL = 1.6 - 1.8$$
$$BMR = 2224.8$$
$$EER = BMR \times PAL$$
$$EER = 2224.8 \times 1.6 \quad \text{to} \quad 2224.8 \times 1.8$$
$$EER = 3559kcal - 4004kcal$$ → Calorie range based on PAL

Rounded to the nearest whole number

W - Weight (kg); **H** - Height (cm); **A** - Age (yrs)
BMR - Basil Metabolic Rate
PAL - Physical Activity Level
EER - Estimated Energy Requirement

The example above shows that this person (weight, height and age values examples only, *please insert your data in their place*), given their age (32yo), weight (104kg), height (189cm), and exertion at work/gym (Moderate) would need to consume between 3559 and 4004 Calories per day.

This person would enter this amount of Calories into apps such as 'MyFitnessPal', 'Chronometer', 'LoseIt', 'LifeSum' or similar to monitor their eating throughout the day. If this person doesn't meet this energy requirement, they may feel exhausted at the end of the day. Exceeding the Calorie range will result in an increase in body fat.

RECOMMENDED DIETARY INTAKE - EER FOR MACRONUTRIENTS

Note that the 'RDI' for Alcohol does not imply that Alcohol is necessary for your health and well being. Alcohol is an energy containing nutrient, and therefore is classed as a Macronutrient. The RDI is a guide provided for anyone CHOOSING to consume Alcohol.

The following Table (*below*) highlighting 'Recommended Dietary Intakes' (RDI) have been adopted from the National Health and Medical Research Council (NHMRC).

MACRONUTRIENT	RDI (PERCENTAGE OF DIET)
Alcohol	RDI = 0 mL. Safe consumption: 2 standard drinks per day, maximum of 4 drinks per day
Carbohydrates	20 - 65% of total EER
Protein	20 - 35% of total EER
Fats	15 - 25% of total EER

CHAPTER 10:

CREATE YOUR OWN MEAL PLAN

In this final chapter we will go through a case study that combines everything in this book and turns it into a Meal Plan. The example given, Jamie, is a guide to help you to build your personalised Meal Plan. All you need to do is substitute your personal information in place of Jamie's.

Please take note that it may be an Offence (illegal) for you to provide Meal Plans to others for the purposes of making money. Fines and possible imprisonment can result. Only a Licensed and/ or Registered Dietician or Nutritionist can legally provide Meal Plans for a fee (money or bartering). The author of this book is a Registered Nutritionist, and a Member of the Nutrition Council of Australia.

CASE STUDY

Step 1. Set a Goal

Jamie is a 32 year old Male, who is 189cm tall, weighs 104kg, is an Office worker who goes to the Gym and engages in Weight training at a moderate intensity 4 - 5 times per week. He is keen to reduce his weight in a healthy way.

To help Jamie reach his weight loss goal, we will combine RDIs for Protein, Carbohydrates, and Fats **(Found in Chapters 3, 4 & 5)**, as well as BMR, PAL and EER **(Found in Chapter 9)**, and take into account the amount of Macronutrients found in foods **(Found in Chapters 3, 4 & 5)** to build a weight loss Meal Plan for Jamie. The information contained in almost all previous chapters will be used.

Step 2. Calculate Your Basil Metabolic Rate (BMR)

From Chapter 9: Energy. Using the Harris-Benedict Formula we will first calculate Jamie's BMR. Then using PAL we will determine how many Calories (EER) he needs to consume to maintain his current weight.

Males $$BMR = 66.44 + (13.75 \times W) + (5.0 \times H) - (6.77 \times A)$$

Females $$BMR = 655.1 + (9.56 \times W) + (1.85 \times H) - (4.68 \times A)$$

W - Weight (kg); **H** - Height (cm); **A** - Age (yrs)

Step 2/3. Calculate Your BMR & Estimated Energy Requirement (EER)

Below. Jamie's Weight, Height and Age has been inserted into the Harris-Benedict formula to determine his current EER. A Physical Activity Factor of 1.6 - 1.8 has been used given Jamie's activity level at the gym. This has been taken from **Chapter 9: Energy**.
If Jamie consumes between 3559 Calories and 4004 Calories based on his moderate intensity activity at the gym, he will maintain his weight of 104kg.

$$BMR = 66.44 + (13.75 \times W) + (5.0 \times H) - (6.77 \times A)$$
$$BMR = 66.44 + (13.75 \times 104) + (5.0 \times 189) - (6.77 \times 32)$$ ⟶ Multiply out each bracket first, then add/ subtract
$$BMR = 66.44 + (1430) + (945) - (216.64)$$
$$BMR = 2224.8$$

$$PAL = 1.6 - 1.8$$
$$BMR = 2224.8$$
$$EER = BMR \times PAL$$
$$EER = 2224.8 \times 1.6 \text{ to } 2224.8 \times 1.8$$
$$EER = 3559kcal - 4004kcal$$ ⟶ Calorie range based on PAL

Rounded to the nearest whole number

W - Weight (kg); **H** - Height (cm); **A** - Age (yrs)
BMR - Basil Metabolic Rate
PAL - Physical Activity Level
EER - Estimated Energy Requirement

\

Step 4: Subtract Enough Calories to Ensure You Lose Weight

In order to actually lose weight, Jamie will have to consume less Calories so that his Energy Balance moves toward a deficit (meaning he will consume less energy than his body actually needs). The body still requires the missing energy, so it will metabolise fat stores in Jamie's body to meet these needs. *Leading to weight loss.*

In **Chapter 5** we discovered that Dietary Fats contain *9 Calories per gram*. The fats stored in Jamie's body, like yours, contains the same amount of energy. **This means that if Jamie wants to lose 1 gram of fat, he will need to create a 9 Calorie deficit.**

If Jamie wants to lose **500 grams of weight per week**. He would need to create a **deficit of 4500 calories**.

If, 1 gram of Fat = 9 calories, then

$9kcal \times 500g = 4500kcal$

$4500kcal \div 7days = 643calorie$ deficit per day

To maintain his weight of 104kg, Jamie would consume: 3559 to 4004 calories per day.
To lose weight, Jamie must subtract 643 calories per day from his diet. So,

$EER = 3559kcal - 4004kcal$

EER = $3559kcal - 643kcal = 2916kcal$ to $4004kcal - 643kcal = 3361kcal$

So Jamie will need to consume between:
2916 kcal to 3361 kcal/ day to lose weight.

IMPORTANT

It is important that you **do not** create an energy deficit that is too large. Doing so will risk slowing/ stalling important biochemical processes in your body from a lack of nutrients. You may have heard that those who 'cut carbs' to lose weight, became grumpy. The biochemical processes that create serotonin and other important neurochemicals require carbohydrates to proceed. A reduction in these neurochemicals can increase your risk of developing mood disorders. **You must consume a varied diet containing every macronutrient.** Of course, Alcohol is optional.

It is highly likely that you will incorporate some level of exercise into your daily routine. All physical activity burns Calories, so any energy that you (or in this case Jamie), uses at the gym must be added to the 643 Calorie deficit we created in his diet (as will you). Depending on how intense Jamie's (or your) workout is at the gym, a 1,000 Calorie deficit can be created very easily. This large deficit will ensure weight loss, while keeping your body fuelled.

Step 5: Calculate Your Macronutrient Requirement

We will now determine how many Calories of each Essential Macronutrient Jamie needs to consume. Half of this table is adapted from **Chapter 9: Energy**.
Given that Jamie is maintaining Moderate Intensity activity, the percentages will be on the higher end of the range. Yours WILL differ depending on your height, weight, activity level and goals.

Given that Jamie is actively going to the gym and engaging in weight training, the Calories requirement will also be on the higher end of the range, in this case 3361 Calories (for weight loss).
The Calories determined in the right-hand column (below) will be used as a guide to build a Meal Plan.

MACRONUTRIENT	RDI (PERCENTAGE OF DIET)	PERCENTAGE USED	MACRONUTRIENT (G) BASED ON 3361KCAL
Alcohol	2 standard drinks per day, maximum of 4 drinks per day	0%	0
Carbohydrates	20 - 65% of total EER	50%	1680 Calores
Protein	20 - 35% of total EER	30%	1008 Calores
Fats	15 - 25% of total EER	20%	672 Calores

This table (below) converts the Calories determined in the right most column of the table *above* into grams of macronutrients that Jamie will need to consume per day.

The table is adapted from Chapter 9: Energy. It shows the amount of Calories in 1 gram of each macronutrient. The Calories above (right column) have been divided by their Calories per gram. To create the right most column in the table below.

ENERGY SOURCE (PER GRAM)	CALORIES (KCAL)	GRAMS OF MACRONUTRIENTS
Fats	9 cal	75g
Alcohol	7 cal	0g
Carbohydrates	4 cal	420g
Protein	4 cal	252g

Now that we know how many grams of each Macronutrient Jamie needs to consume, we can use this information along with the tables found in **Chapters 1 - 9** to build a Meal Plan geared toward weight loss.
Remember that the goal is to get close to these Macronutrients. Sometimes they will be off (under/ over). But what matters most is the amount of Calories that you consume. Energy Balance is the be all end all of weight loss.

EXAMPLE CALCULATION

Jamie will need to consume approximately 1680 calories in Carbohydrates.
Carbohydrates have 4 calories per gram. So,

$1680kcal \div 4kcal = 420g$ Carbohydrates per day

So Jamie will need to consume:
420g of Carbohydrates per day.

Step 6: Estimate Your Fluid (Water) Requirement

From **Chapter 6**, your estimated fluid intake - Water (EFR) can be calculated. Substitute your own values.

Jamie's Estimated Fluid (Water) Requirement (EPR) based on his activity level, and guidelines found in **Chapter 6: Hydration**

$EFR = 30mL - 35mL/$ kg of body weight
$30mL \times 104kg = 3120mL$
$35mL \times 104kg = 3640mL$

So Jamie will need to consume between:
3120mL and 3640mL water/ day

Step 7: Build Your Meal Plan

Use the tables in **Chapters 2 - 7** to create your meal plan. Here (*below*), foods have been chosen to divide up the Calories and macronutrients that Jamie needs to consume over 5 meals. You can choose to divide your energy requirements (meals) as you wish. It is important to pay attention to RDI values and percentages throughout this book to ensure your intake of Macro & Micro nutrients is adequate.

MEAL 1: BREAKFAST				
FOOD	CARBOHYDRATES (G)	PROTEIN (G)	FATS (G)	ENERGY (KCAL)
3x Eggs	1.3g	14.8g	17.1g	250 Cal
3x Multigrain toast	52.2g	10g	3.3g	291 Cal
1x Apple	14.6g	0.4g	0g	45 Cal
100g Avocado	1g	4g	16g	204 Cal
Large Cappuccino (400mL)	10.1g	6.8g	6.8g	124 Cal
TOTAL	79.2g	35.8g	43.2g	**914 Cal**

MEAL 2 : SNACK				
FOOD	CARBOHYDRATES (G)	PROTEIN (G)	FATS (G)	ENERGY (KCAL)
1x Med Banana	21.8g	19.g	0.1g	100 Cal
170g Strawberries	16.8g	13.8g	0.3g	127 Cal
30g Honey	24.7g	0g	0g	91 Cal
150g Greek yogurt	4.4g	15.9g	0g	80 Cal
TOTAL	67.7g	31.6g	0.4g	**398 Cal**

MEAL 3: LUNCH				
FOOD	**CARBOHYDRATES (G)**	**PROTEIN (G)**	**FATS (G)**	**ENERGY (KCAL)**
150g Pasta	36.9g	7.7g	1.2g	207 Cal
150g Chicken (Skinless)	0g	33.6g	2.4g	156 Cal
125g Pasta sauce	11.1g	1.6g	0.1g	56 Cal
1 Cup Mixed salad	8.6g	1.8g	0.3g	44 Cal
2 Tbs Parmesan cheese	0g	6.1g	5g	70 Cal
TOTAL	56.6g	50.8g	9g	**533 Cal**

MEAL 4: SNACK				
FOOD	**CARBOHYDRATES (G)**	**PROTEIN (G)**	**FATS (G)**	**ENERGY (KCAL)**
2x Cups Fruit Salad	30g	2.8g	0.8g	148 Cal
50g Mixed Nuts	12.7g	8.7g	25.8g	297 Cal
Large Cappuccino (400mL)	10.1g	6.8g	6.8g	124 Cal
TOTAL	52.8g	18.3g	33.4g	**569 Cal**

MEAL 5: DINNER				
FOOD	**CARBOHYDRATES (G)**	**PROTEIN (G)**	**FATS (G)**	**ENERGY (KCAL)**
150g Lean beef	0g	37.7g	19.4g	336 Cal
2x Cups Broccoli	1.2g	14.4g	1g	96 Cal
1x Cup Mash Potatoes	22.9g	5.3g	11.6g	222 Cal
1x Cup Mixed salad	8.6g	1.8g	0.3g	44 Cal
2 Tbs Tomato sauce	7.6g	0.4g	0.1g	110 Cal
1x Bottle full strength beer (4.8% Alc. Vol)	10.1g	0g	0g	136 cal
TOTAL	47.3g	60g	32.3g	**944 Cal**

TOTAL MACRONUTRIENTS & CALORIES FROM MEAL PLAN				
MACRONUTRIENT	**MACRONUTRIENT GOAL (GRAMS)**	**CALORIES GOAL**	**MACRONUTRIENT ACTUAL FROM MEAL PLAN**	**CALORIES FROM MEAL PLAN (KCAL)**
Carbohydrates	420g	1680 Calores	303g	1212
Protein	252g	1008 Calores	196g	784
Fats	75g	672 Calores	118g	1062
TOTALS	-	**3360 Calories**	-	3058

Jamie's total Calorie intake for this Meal Plan comes to approximately 3360 Calories from a target of 3361 Calories.

It is very important that you consume the amount of food that your body needs, rather than just using this example as your Meal Plan. This example is provided to illustrate how to build a Meal Plan of your own based on your body, lifestyle and goals. Your meal plan must stay within your Calorie intake for weight loss. Do your best to meet the energy (Calorie) target.

You will note that the Meal Plan shows an of skew Macronutrient intake, this is by design. It has been created this way to illustrate to you that attempting to create a perfect meal plan is not the point. The idea is to choose healthier options, and to stay within your Calorie intake. Do your best to choose a variety of foods to meet your Macronutrient requirements. Do the best you can with the budget you have.

REFERENCES

1. American Heart Association. (2018). Added Sugars. (online) Available at: http://www.heart.org/ HEARTORG/HealthyLiving/ HealthyEating/Nutrition/Added-Sugars_UCM_305858_Article.jsp#. Wv0D4C9L1TZ

2. Aronson, D. (2009). Cortisol — Its Role in Stress, Inflammation, and Indications for Diet Therapy. [online] Today's Dietitian. Available at: https://www.todaysdietitian.com/newarchives/111609p38.shtml

3. Aune, D., Giovannucci, E., Boffetta, P., Fadnes, L., Keum, N., Norat, T., Greenwood, D., Riboli, E., Vatten, L. and Tonstad, S. (2017). Fruit and vegetable intake and the risk of cardiovascular disease, total cancer and all-cause mortality—a systematic review and dose-response meta-analysis of prospective studies. International Journal of Epidemiology, 46(3), pp.1029-1056.

4. Australian Bureau of Statistics. (2016). 4364.0.55.012 - Australian Health Survey: Consumption of Food Groups from the Australian Dietary Guidelines, 2011-12. [online] Available at: http://www.abs.gov.au/ ausstats/abs@.nsf/Lookup/by%20Subject/ 4364.0.55.012~2011-12~Main%20Features~Lean%20meats%20 and%20alternatives~13

5. Australian Bureau of Statistics. (2017). 4364.0.55.011 - Australian Health Survey: Consumption of added sugars, 2011-12. [online] Available at: http://www.abs.gov.au/ausstats/abs@.nsf/Lookup/by%20 Subject/ 4364.0.55.011~2011-12~Main%20Features~Consumption%20of%20Added%20Sugars%20-%20 A%20comparison%20of%201995%20to%202011-12~20

6. Berg, J., Tymoczko, J. and Stryer, L. (2002). Triacylglycerols Are Highly Concentrated Energy Stores. [online] Ncbi.nlm.nih.gov. Available at: https://www.ncbi.nlm.nih.gov/books/NBK22369/

7. Collado, M., Isolauri, E., Salminen, S. and Sanz, Y. (2009). The Impact of Probiotic on Gut Health. Current Drug Metabolism, 10(1), pp.68-78.

8. Dehghan, M., Mente, A., Zhang, X., Swaminathan, S., Li, W. and Mohan, V. (2017). Associations of fats and carbohydrate intake with cardiovascular disease and mortality in 18 countries from five continents (PURE): a prospective cohort study. The Lancet, 390(10107), pp.2050-2062.

9. Ekinci, E., Clarke, S., Thomas, M., Moran, J., Cheong, K., MacIsaac, R. and Jerums, G. (2011). Dietary Salt Intake and Mortality in Patients With Type 2 Diabetes. Diabetes Care, 34(3), pp.703-709.

10. Eat For Health. (2017). Discretionary Food And Drink Choices. (online) Available: https://www.eatforhealth.gov.au/food-essentials/discretionary-food-and-drink-choices

11. Foundation for Alcohol Research & Education. (2019). Australian Drinking Guidelines. [online] Available at: http://fare.org.au/ resources/australian-drinking-guidelines/

12. Gastrointestinal Society. (2018). Physical Activity and GI Health. [online] Available at: https://www.badgut.org/information-centre/a-z-digestive-topics/physical-activity-and-gi- health/

13. Goodson, A. (2018). Top 8 Vitamins and Nutrients for Healthy, Strong Nails. [online] Health Line. Available at: https:// www.healthline.com/nutrition/vitamins-for-nails

14. Hadhazy, A. (2019). Think Twice: How the Gut's "Second Brain" Influences Mood and Well-Being. [online] Scientific American. Available at: https://www.scientificamerican.com/article/gut-second-brain/

15. Healthline. (2018). How Many Carbs Should You Eat Per Day to Lose Weight?. [online] Available at: https://www.healthline.com/nutrition/how-many-carbs-per-day-to-lose-weight#section1

16. Health.qld.gov.au. (2017). Estimating energy, protein & fluid requirements for adult clinical conditions. [online] Available at: https://www.health.qld.gov.au/__data/assets/pdf_file/0022/144175/est_rqts.pdf

17. Healsop, M. (2012). The Health Risks Associated with Prolonged Sedentary Behaviour: A Systematic Review. Joanna Briggs Institute, [online] The University of Adelaide. Available at: https://digital.library. adelaide.edu.au/dspace/bitstream/ 2440/74097/8/02whole.pdf

18. Heart Foundation. (n.d.). Dietary Fat and Heart Healthy Eating. [online]
Available at: https://www.heartfoundation.org.au/images/uploads/main/For_professionals/Dietary_Fats_Position_Statement_2017.pdf

19. Heart Foundation. (2018). Saturated and Trans Fats. (online) Available at: https://www.heartfoundation. org.au/healthy-eating/food-and-nutrition/fats-and-cholesterol/saturated-and-trans-fat

20. Hjalmarsdottir, F. (2018). 17 Science-Based Benefits of Omega-3 Fatty Acids. [online] Health Line. Available at: https://www.healthline.com/nutrition/17-health-benefits-of-omega-3#section13

21. Hoffman, J. and Falvo, M. (2004). Protein - Which is best?. Journal of Sports Science and Medicine, 3(3), pp.118-130.

22. Holtmann, G. and Enck, P. (2008). Stress and Gastrointestinal Motility in Humans: A Review of the Literature. Neurogastroenterology & Motility, 3(4), pp.245-254.

23. Institute of Medicine. 2005. Dietary Reference Intakes for Energy, Carbohydrate, Fiber, Fat, Fatty Acids, Cholesterol, Protein, and Amino Acids. Washington, DC: The National Academies Press. https://doi.org/10.17226/10490

24. Jäger, R., Kerksick, C., Campbell, B., Cribb, P., Wells, S., Skwiat, T., Purpura, M., Ziegenfuss, T., Ferrando, A., Arent, S., Smith-Ryan, A., Stout, J., Arciero, P., Ormsbee, M., Taylor, L., Wilborn, C., Kalman, D., Kreider, R., Willoughby, D., Hoffman, J., Krzykowski, J. and Antonio, J. (2017). International Society of Sports Nutrition Position Stand: protein and exercise. Journal of the International Society of Sports Nutrition, 14(1).

25. Jandhyala, S. (2015). Role of the normal gut microbiota. World Journal of Gastroenterology, 21(29), p.8787.

26. Jay R. Hoffman, M. (2019). Protein - Which is Best?. [online] Jssm.org. Available at: https://www.jssm.org/hf.php?id=jssm-03-118.xml

27. Kapoor, R. and Huang, Y. (2006). Gamma linolenic acid: an antiinflammatory omega-6 fatty acid. Current Pharmaceutical Biotechnology, 7(6), pp.531-4.

28. Kiela, P. and Ghishan, F. (2016). Physiology of Intestinal Absorption and Secretion. Best Practice & Research Clinical Gastroenterology, 30(2), pp.145-159.

29. Kim, D. and Camilleri, M. (2000). Serotonin: a mediator of the brain-gut connection. The American Journal of Gastroenterology, 95(10), pp.2698-2709.

30. Kim, E. and Rhee, P. (2012). How to Interpret a Functional or Motility Test - Colon Transit Study. Journal of Neurogastroenterology and Motility, 18(1), pp.94-99.

31. Liu, A., Ford, N., Hu, F., Zelman, K., Mozaffarian, D. and Kris-Etherton, P. (2017). A healthy approach to dietary fats: understanding the science and taking action to reduce consumer confusion. Nutrition Journal, 16(1).

32. Manners, D. (2010). What Causes Constipation?. [online] Food Intol.
Available at: https://www.foodintol.com/what-causes-constipation

33. Martini, F. and Nath, J. (2009). Fundamentals of anatomy & physiology. 8th ed. San Francisco: Pearson Education Inc.

34. Mentzer, A. (2018). Long-Term Risks of Low Fiber. [online] Healthy Eating.
Available at: https://healthyeating.sfgate.com/longterm-risks-low-fiber-1267.html

35. Miglio, C., Chiavaro, E., Visconti, A., Fogliano, V. and Pellegrini, N. (2008). Effects of Different Cooking Methods on Nutritional and Physicochemical Characteristics of Selected Vegetables. Journal of Agricultural and Food Chemistry, 56(1), pp.139-147.

36. Miglio, C., Chiavaro, E., Visconti, A., et al. (2008). Effects of Different Cooking Methods On Nutritional and Physicochemical Characteristics of Selected Vegetables. Journal of Agricultural and Food Chemistry, vol. 56 (1), pp. 139-47. URL: https://pubs.acs.org/doi/abs/10.1021/jf072304b

37. Mozaffarian, D. (2006). Trans fatty acids – Effects on systemic inflammation and endothelial function. Atherosclerosis Supplements, 7(2), pp.29-32.

38. National Health and Medical Research Council (2014). Nutrient Reference Values for Australia and New Zealand: Macronutrient Balance. URL: https://www.nrv.gov.au/chronic-disease/macronutrient-balance

39. National Health and Medical Research Council. (2009). Alcohol. [online]
Available at: https://nhmrc.gov.au/health-advice/alcohol

40. National Health and Medical Research Council (2017). Nutrient Reference Values for Australia and New Zealand: Dietary Energy. URL: https://www.nrv.gov.au/dietary-energy

41. NSW Ministry of Health. (2013). NSW Healthy Eating and Active Living Strategy. [online]
Available at: https://www.health.nsw.gov.au/heal/publications/nsw-healthy-eating-strategy.pdf

42. Nutrient Reference Values. (2014). Water. [online] Available at: https://www.nrv.gov.au/nutrients/water

43. Nutrient Reference Values. (2014). Dietary Fibre. [online] Available at: https://www.nrv.gov.au/nutrients/dietary-fibre

44. Nutrient Reference Values. (2014). Protein. [online] Available at: https://www.nrv.gov.au/nutrients/protein

45. Nutrient Reference Values. (2014). Carbohydrates [online] Available at: https://www.nrv.gov.au/nutrients/carbohydrates

46. Nutrient Reference Values. (2017). Nutrients. [online] Available at: https://www.nrv.gov.au/nutrients

47. Nutrition Australia. (2016). VHEE fruit & veg resource hub. [online]
Available at: http://www.nutritionaustralia.org/vic/resource/vhee-fruit-veg-resource-hub

48. Pannemans D.L.E., Wagenmakers A.J.M., Westerterp K.R., Schaafsma G., Halliday D. (1998) Effect of protein source

49. Phillips, S., Chevalier, S. and Leidy, H., 2016. Protein "requirements" beyond the RDA: implications for optimizing health. Applied Physiology, Nutrition, and Metabolism, 41(5), pp.565-572.

50. Renee, J. (2018). Recommended Amount of Unsaturated Fat per Day. [online] SF Gate.
Available at: https://healthyeating.sfgate.com/recommended-amount-unsaturated-fat-per-day-6385. html

51. Schomburg, I., Chang, A., Placzek, S., Söhngen, C., Rother, M., Lang, M., Munaretto, C., Ulas, S., Stelzer, M., Grote, A., Scheer, M. and Schomburg, D. (2012). BRENDA in 2013: integrated reactions, kinetic data, enzyme function data, improved disease classification: new options and contents in BRENDA. Nucleic Acids Research, 41(D1), pp.D764-D772.

52. Schönfeld, P. and Wojtczak, L. (2016). Short- and medium-chain fatty acids in energy metabolism: the cellular perspective. Journal of Lipid Research, 57(6), pp.943-954.

53. The Heart Foundation. (n.d.). Saturated and trans fat. [online]
Available at: https://www.heartfoundation.org.au/healthy-eating/food-and-nutrition/fats-and- cholesterol/saturated-and-trans-fat

54. USDA Food Composition Databases. (2018). Food Composition Databases Show Nutrients List. [online] Available at: https://ndb.nal.usda.gov/ndb/nutrients/report?nutrient1=203&nutrient2 =&nutrient3=&&max=25&subset=0&offset=0&sort=c&totCount=7524&measureby=g

55. Vighi, G., Marcucci, F., Sensi, L., Di Cara, G. and Frati, F. (2008). Allergy and the gastrointestinal system. Clinical & Experimental Immunology, 153, pp.3-6.

56. World Health Organization. (2018). Increasing fruit and vegetable consumption to reduce the risk of noncommunicable diseases. [online] Available at: http://www.who.int/elena/titles/fruit_vegetables_ ncds/en/

57. World Health Organisation. (n.d.). Micronutrients. [online]
Available at: https://www.who.int/nutrition/topics/micronutrients/en/

58. World Health Organisation. (2019). Promoting fruit and vegetable consumption around the world. [online] Available at: https://www.who.int/dietphysicalactivity/fruit/en/

59. www.heart.org. (2019). Added Sugars. [online] Available at: http://www.heart.org/HEARTORG/ HealthyLiving/HealthyEating/Nutrition/Added-Sugars_UCM_305858_Article.jsp#.WaU1o1QjHIU

Made in the USA
Monee, IL
04 November 2026

67388676R00026